HEPATITIS C

A complete guide on Hepatitis C, Symptoms, Causes, Risk Factors, Medical prescriptions and Cure: Also a comprehensive guide for Health Practitioners, Medical Professionals or Caregivers

Dr. Kate D. Martins

Introduction

The History of Hepatitis C

During the 1970s, Harvey J. Alter, Head of the Infectious Disease Section in the Department of Transfusion Medicine at the National Institutes of Health showed how most post-transfusion hepatitis cases were not because of hepatitis A or B viruses. Notwithstanding this discovery, worldwide research endeavors to identify the infection, at first called non-A, non-B hepatitis (NANBH), failed for the following 10 years.

Michael Houghton, Qui-Lim Choo, and George Kuo worked with Daniel W. in 1987 at Chiron Corporation at the Centers for Disease Control and Prevention, using an original subatomic cloning way to deal with identifying the obscure organism and conduct a diagnostic examination. In 1988, Alter affirmed the infection by checking its presence in a board of NANBH sample and specimen, and Chiron reported its disclosure at a Washington, DC Public interview in May 1988.

At that point, Chiron was in talks with the Japanese health service to sell a biotech version of the hepatitis B immunization vaccine. At the same time, Emperor Hirohito had developed cancer and required various blood transfusions. Chiron's experimental NANBH test received a screening order from the Japanese health ministry. The term "Hepatitis C" was first used in November 1988 by Diagnostic Systems KK, a Japanese marketing subsidiary of Chiron, in Tokyo news reports about the testing of the emperor's blood. In November 1988, Chiron made $60 million annually by selling a screening order to the Japanese health ministry. Nonetheless, in light of the fact that Chiron had not distributed any of its examination and research and didn't make a culture model accessible to different scientists to confirm Chiron's discovery, hepatitis C procured the nickname **"The emperor's New Infection"**

"The "discovery" of HCV was reported in two Science articles in April 1989. Chiron petitioned for a few licenses on the infection and its diagnosis. A pending patent application by the CDC was dropped in 1990 after Chiron paid $1.9 million to the CDC and $337,500 to Bradley. In 1994, Bradley sued Chiron, looking to invalidate the patent, have himself included as a co-inventor, and get damages and royalty pay. The court disallowed him, which was supported on claim in 1998.In view of the special sub-atomic "isolation" of the hepatitis C virus or infection, in spite of the fact that Houghton and Kuo's group at Chiron had identified strong bio-chemicals for the infection and the test proved to be successful at diminishing instances of post-transfusion hepatitis, the existence of a

hepatitis C infection was instantly inferred. In 1992, the San Francisco Chronicle revealed that the infection had never been tested and observed under an electron microscope. In 1997, the American FDA endorsed the principal hepatitis C drug based on a proxy marker called "Sustained Virological Reaction." Accordingly, the pharmaceutical industry formed a cross country organization of "Astro-Turf" patient support groups to bring issues to light (and feeling of fear) toward the disease.

In 2005, a Japanese team was able to propagate a molecular clone known as Huh7 in a cell culture and finally "discovered" hepatitis C. This disclosure empowered appropriate portrayal of the viral molecule and quick research into the development of protease inhibitors supplanting early interferon treatment. The first of these, sofosbuvir, was approved on December 6, 2013. These medications are marketed as "cures;" in any case, since they were endorsed based on surrogate markers and not clinical endpoints, for example, prolonging life or improving liver wellbeing, numerous specialists question their value.

After blood screening started, a hepatitis C predominance was found in Egypt, which guaranteed 6,000,000 people were infected by unsterile needles in a late 1970s mass chemotherapy Campaign to take out schistosomiasis (snail fever).

On October 5, 2020, Houghton and Alter, along with Charles M. Rice was given the Nobel Prize in Physiology or Medicine for their efforts.

Chapter 1

An Overview of Hepatitis C

Hepatitis C is an irresistible (infectious) disease brought about by the hepatitis C virus (HCV) that principally influences the liver; it is a kind of viral hepatitis.

During the infection's early phase, individuals frequently have little or no symptoms. Early signs and symptoms can include fever, stomach pain, yellow touched skin and dark urine. The infection continues in the liver, becoming persistent, in around 70% of those at first infected. Over numerous years notwithstanding, it frequently prompts liver infection and frequent cirrhosis. Now and again, those with cirrhosis will foster serious complications like liver failure, dilated veins, in the throat and stomach, liver cancer.

HCV is spread fundamentally by blood-to-blood contact related with injection drug use, ineffectively sanitized clinical equipment or tools, needle stick wounds in medical care, and transfusions. In areas where blood screening has been carried out, the great risk of contracting HCV from a transfusion has dropped considerably to 1 per every two million. HCV may likewise be spread from a contaminated or infected mother to her child during birth. However, It is not spread through breast milk, food, water or usual contact like kissing, hugging and sharing food with an infected individual. It is one of five known hepatitis infections: A, B, C, D, and E.[7] Diagnosis is by blood testing to search for either antibodies to the virus or viral RNA.

In the US, screening for HCV infection is prescribed in all grown-ups aged 18 to 79 years old. There is no immunization or vaccine against hepatitis C.

Prevention incorporates harm decrease endeavors among individuals who inject drugs, testing donated blood, and treatment of individuals with infection. Chronic contamination can be cured over 95% of the time with antiviral drugs, for example, sofosbuvir or simeprevir.

Peginterferon and ribavirin were former generation medicines that demonstrated to be successful in <50% of cases and caused more harmful side effects. 2015 variant. While access to the recent medicines was costly, by 2022 costs had dropped in numerous nations (principally lower-income countries) because of the presentation of generic forms of medicines. But people who foster cirrhosis or liver cancer, in most cases might require a liver transplant.

Hepatitis C is one of the main explanations behind liver transplantation, however the infection normally reoccur after transplantation. An expected 58 million individuals overall were diagnosed or infected with hepatitis C in 2019. In addition, hepatitis C-related liver cancer and cirrhosis accounted for approximately 290,000 deaths in 2019. The presence of hepatitis C - initially recognizable just as a kind of non-A non-B hepatitis - was recommended during the 1970s and proven in 1989. Hepatitis C infects just humans and chimpanzees.

Chapter 2

Signs and symptoms

Acute Infection

An acute symptom is developed in some 20% of those infected. When this happens, it is by and large 4-12 weeks following contamination (however it might take from 2 weeks to a half year for intense signs and symptoms to appear).

Symptoms are for the most part little or unclear, and may incorporate exhaustion, fever, muscle or joint pain, nausea and vomiting, stomach pain, decrease in appetite and weight reduction, jaundice (happens in ~25% of those tainted), dull pee, and earth shaded stools.[Acute liver failure brought on by hepatitis C is extremely uncommon. Symptoms and laboratory results that point to liver disease should prompt additional tests, which can help diagnose hepatitis C early on.

Following the acute stage, the contamination might determine suddenly in 10-50% of affected individuals; this happens all the more much of the time in young people and females.

Chronic Infection

Around 70% of those exposed to the infection foster a chronic infection. This is characterized as the presence of noticeable viral replication for not less than 7 months. However most experience negligible or Symptoms during the first few decades of a persistent infection, chronic hepatitis C can be related with fatigue and little mental problems. Following quite a long while, chronic infection might cause cirrhosis or liver cancer. The liver proteins estimated from blood tests are ordinary in 7-53%. (High levels show liver cells are being harmed by the infection or other illness). Late backslides after cure have been accounted for, however these can be challenging to differentiate from reinfection.

Fatty changes to the liver happen in about a portion of the number of those infected and are generally present before cirrhosis develops. Typically (80% of the time) this change affects under 33% of the liver. Hepatitis C accounts for 25% of hepatocellular carcinoma and 27% of cirrhosis cases worldwide. Around 10-30% of those infected foster cirrhosis for more than 30 years. Alcoholics, male sex, and people who are also infected with hepatitis B, , or HIV are more likely to develop cirrhosis. In those with hepatitis C, alcohol in excess builds the risk of creating cirrhosis 5-fold. The individuals who developed cirrhosis have a 20X more serious risk of hepatocellular carcinoma.

This change happens at a pace of 1-3% per year. Being infected with hepatitis B notwithstanding hepatitis C increases this hazard further.

Ascites—

An accumulation of fluid in the abdomen—easy bruising or bleeding, varices—enlarged veins, especially in the stomach and esophagus—jaundice, and a cognitive impairment syndrome known as hepatic encephalopathy—are all symptoms of liver cirrhosis. Ascites happens at some stage in the greater part of the people who have a constant infection.

Extrahepatic difficulties

The most widely usual issue because of hepatitis C yet not including the liver is mixed cryoglobulinemia (normally the type II structure) - an irritation of little and medium-sized blood vessels. Hepatitis C is likewise connected with immune system problems, for example, Sjögren's disorder, lichen planus, a low platelet count, porphyria cutanea tarda, necrolytic acral erythema, insulin opposition, diabetes mellitus, diabetic nephropathy, immune system thyroiditis, and B-cell lymphoproliferative disorders. 20-30% of individuals infected have rheumatoid factors - a kind of antibody. Potential affiliations include Hyde's prurigo

nodularis and membranoproliferative glomerulonephritis. Cardiomyopathy with related abnormal heart rhythms has additionally been reported. An assortment of focal and fringe sensory system issues has been reported. Chronic infection by all accounts is related to a high risk of pancreatic cancer. Individuals might encounter different problems in the mouth, for example, dryness, salivary pipe stones, and crusted injuries around the mouth.
Occult disease

Individuals who have been infected with hepatitis C might seem to clear the infection however remain infected. The infection isn't perceivable with traditional testing yet can be found with ultra-sensitive tests. The first technique of detection was by exhibiting the *viral genome inside liver biopsies, but newer strategies include an immunizer test for the infection's center protein and the recognition of the viral genome after first focusing the viral particles by ultracentrifugation. A type of disease with persistently high serum liver enzymes but without antibodies to hepatitis C has likewise been reported. This structure is known as cryptogenic occult infection.*

A few clinical pictures have been related to this kind of infection. It very well might be found in individuals with anti-hepatitis-C antibodies yet with typical serum levels of liver chemicals; in antibody-negative individuals with progressing high liver enzymes of obscure reason; in healthy populaces without proof of liver sickness;

and in groups in danger of HCV disease, that include those on hemodialysis or relatives of individuals with occult HCV. The medical relevance of this type of contamination is under investigation. The outcomes of occult disease have all the earmarks of being less extreme than with chronic infection yet can fluctuate from little to hepatocellular carcinoma.

The pace of occult disease in those obviously cured is dubious yet has all the signs of being low. 40% of those with hepatitis yet with both negative hepatitis C serology and the absence of viral genome in the serum have hepatitis C infection in the liver on biopsy. How usually this happens in kids is yet to be known.

Chapter 3

Transfusion

Percutaneous contact with infected blood is responsible for most infections; notwithstanding, the technique for transmission is emphatically subject to both geographic area and the status of the economy. For sure, the essential course of transmission in the world is injection drug use, while in the developed world, the fundamental strategies are blood transfusion and unsafe clinical procedures. The reason for transmission is still obscure or unknown in 20% of cases; notwithstanding, a considerable lot of these are accepted to be accounted for by injection drug use.

Drug use

Infusion or injection drug use (IDU) is a great risk factor for hepatitis C in many parts of the world. Of 77 nations explored, 25 (counting in the US) were found to have a prevalence of hepatitis C of 60-80% among individuals who use injection drugs. Twelve nations had rates more noteworthy than 80%. It is believed that ten million intravenous drug users are diagnosed with hepatitis C; China (1.6 million), the US (1.5 million), and Russia (1.3 million) have the most absolute totals. The occurrence of hepatitis C among jail detainees (inmates) in the US is 10-20% of that observed in general populations; this has been ascribed to high-risk behavior in penitentiaries or prisons like IDU and tattooing with non-sterile tools. Shared intranasal drug use may likewise be a great risk factor.

Health Exposure

Blood transfusion, transfusion of blood items, or organ transplant without HCV screening has huge dangers of infection. The US founded universal screening in 1992, and Canada did the same in 1990. This greatly reduced from between one out of 10,000 to one of every 10,000,000 for each unit of blood. This low risk remains as there is a time of around 11-70 days between the potential blood donors contacting hepatitis C and the blood's testing positive relying upon the method. A few nations don't screen for hepatitis C due to the cost.

The people who have encountered a needle stick injury from somebody who was HCV positive have about a 1.8% chance of being infected by the disease themselves. The risk is more prominent on the off chance that the needle is empty and the stabbing is deep. There is a risk from mucosal openings to blood, however this risk is low, and there is no risk or danger assuming that blood exposure happens on flawless and intact skin.

Clinic equipment has likewise been documented as a method for transmission of hepatitis C, including reuse of syringe or needles, multiple used prescription vials, infusion packs, and inappropriately disinfected surgical tools, among others. Impediments in the execution and requirement of high standard precautions in both private and public and dental offices are known to have been the essential cause of the spread of HCV in Egypt, the country that had the highest rate of disease on the planet in 2012, and at present.

Sex

Sexual transmission of hepatitis C is uncommon. Studies looking at the risk of HCV transmission between heterosexuals, when one is infected and the other isn't, have found extremely low risks. Sexual practices that include more high levels of injury to the anogenital mucosa, like anal penetrative sex, or that happen when there is a simultaneous physically sexually transmitted disease, including HIV or genital ulceration, present bigger risks. The US Department of Veterans affairs prescribes condom use to forestall hepatitis C transmission in those with numerous sexual partners, however not those in a relationship with one partner.

Body adjustment and Modification

Tattooing is related to a two to triple rate of increased risk of hepatitis C. This could be because of either inappropriately disinfected equipment or contamination of the colors being used. Tattoos or piercings done either before the mid-1980s, "underground", or

Nonprofessionally are of specific concern, since sterile procedures in such settings are not available. The risk likewise seems, by all accounts, to be greater for bigger tattoos. It is assessed that almost 50% of jail detainees share unsterilized tattooing tools. It is uncommon for tattoos in an authorized or licensed office to be connected directly with HCV infection.

Shared individual things

Personal stuff like razors, toothbrushes, and manicuring or pedicuring tools can be sullied or contaminated with blood. Sharing such things might possibly lead to the exposure of HCV. Fitting caution ought to be taken with respect to any ailment that results in bleedings, like cuts and sores. HCV isn't spread through contact like kissing, hugging or sharing eating, cooking or kitchen utensils, nor is it communicated through food or water.

Mother-to-child transmission

Mother-to-child transmission of hepatitis C happens in less than 10% of pregnancies. There are no confirmed measures that modify this risk. It isn't clear when transmission happens during pregnancy, yet it might happen both during gestation and perhaps at delivery. A long labor is related with a more serious risk of transmission. There is no proof that breastfeeding spreads HCV; Regardless, to be mindful, an infected mother is encouraged to abstain from breastfeeding assuming her areolas or nipples are broken and bleeding, or on the other hand assuming that her viral loads are high.

Chapter 4

Diagnosis

HCV antibody enzyme immunoassay (ELISA), recombinant immunoblot assay, and quantitative HCV RNA polymerase chain reaction (PCR) are three diagnostic test for hepatitis C. HCV RNA can be detected by PCR regularly one to about fourteen days after being infected, while antibodies can take significantly longer to develop and be detected.

Diagnosing patients is by and large a difficult thing as patients with acute disease for the most part present with little, vague influenza like symptoms, while the change from acute to chronic is sub-clinical. Chronic hepatitis C is characterized as a disease with the hepatitis C infection persevering for over half a year in view of the presence of its RNA. Chronic infection on the other hand is regularly asymptomatic during the initial phase and decades, and consequently are most normally found following the examination of high liver enzyme levels or during a standard screening of high-risk people. Testing can't differentiate chronic and Acute infections. Diagnosis in newborn children is troublesome as maternal antibodies might endure for up to eighteen months.

Serology

Hepatitis C testing regularly starts with blood testing to detect the presence of antibodies to the HCV, utilizing an enzyme immunoassay. On the off chance that this test is positive, a confirmatory test is performed to check the immunoassay and to decide the viral load. A recombinant immunoblot measure is used to check the immunoassay and the viral load by a HCV RNA polymerase chain reaction. In the event that there is no RNA and the immunoblot is positive, it implies that the individual tested had a past disease, however cleared it either with treatment or immediately; if the immunoblot is negative, it implies that the immunoassay was wrong. It requires around two months before the immunoassay will test positive. Various tests are accessible as the reason behind point-of-care testing (POCT), which can give results in 30 minutes.

During the initial stages of the infection, liver enzymes vary, but they typically begin to rise seven weeks after infection. The height of liver enzymes doesn't intently follow sickness severity.

Liver biopsies are used to decide the level of liver damage present; nonetheless, there are risks from the procedure. The normal changes seen are lymphocytes inside the parenchyma, lymphoid follicles in portal ternion, and changes to the bile ducts. There are various blood tests accessible that attempt to detect the level of hepatic fibrosis and lighten the requirement for biopsy.

Screening

It is naturally believed that five-fifty percent of those contaminated in the US and Canada know about their status. Routine evaluation or screening for those between the ages of 18 and 79 was suggested by the US Preventive Task force in the year 2020. Already, testing was suggested for those at high risk, including injection drug users, the individuals who have received blood transfusion before the year 1992, the people who have been incarcerated, those on long haul hemodialysis, and those with tattoos.

Screening is additionally suggested for those with higher liver catalyst (enzymes), as this is every now and again the main indication and sign of constant hepatitis. As of the year 2012, Centers for Disease Control and Prevention (CDC) suggests a single evaluating test for those given birth to somewhere in the range of 1945 and 1965. In Canada, a one-time screening is suggested for those given birth to somewhere in the range of 1945 and 1975.

Chapter 5

Prevention & Treatments

How is Hepatitis C acquired?

Hepatitis C infection is found in the blood of individuals with HCV disease. It enters the body through contact with blood.

Until blood tests for HCV were created (around 1992), individuals typically got hepatitis C from blood items or blood *transfusions. Now that blood items and blood are tried and tested for HCV, this is presently not the run of the mill method for disease.*

Prevention

<u>Hepatitis C vaccine</u>

Starting around 2022, no vaccine could make one immune against contracting hepatitis C. A blend of harm reduction techniques, for example, the provision of new syringe and needles and treatment of substance use, diminishes the risk of hepatitis C in individuals using injection drugs by around 75%. The screening of blood donors is very vital and significant at a public level, as is submitting to universal insurances within medical services facilities. In nations where there is a lacking supply of sterilized needles, drugs ought to be given orally as opposed to through infusion and injection (when possible). Recent exploration additionally proposes that treating individuals with active disease, in this manner lessening the potential for transmission, might be a compelling preventive measure.

Treatment

1. *Those with chronic hepatitis C are encouraged to keep away from alcohol or liquor and meds that are harmful to the liver.*

2. *Due to the increased risk of infection, they should also be vaccinated against hepatitis A and hepatitis B.*

3. *The use of acetaminophen is by and large viewed as safe at lower doses.*

4. *Nonsteroidal anti-inflammatory drugs (NSAIDs) are not suggested in those with advanced liver disease because of an expanded risk of bleeding.*

5. *Ultrasound observation for hepatocellular carcinoma is suggested in those with cirrhosis.*

6. *Coffee has been related with a [vague] or slower pace of liver scarring in those diagnosed with HCV.*

Medications

Ribavirin

Over 95% of chronic cases clear with treatment. Treatment with antiviral medication is suggested for all individuals with demonstrated chronic hepatitis C who are not at high risk of death from other causes.

The severity of liver scarring determines which patients face the greatest risk of complications and should be treated first. The underlying suggested treatment relies upon the kind of hepatitis C infection, assuming the individual has gotten past hepatitis C treatment, and whether the individual has cirrhosis.

According to testing for virus particles in the blood of patients, direct-acting antivirals are the preferred treatment.

Surgery

Cirrhosis because of hepatitis C is a typical justification behind liver transplantation, however the infection generally (80-90% of cases) repeats afterwards.

Disease of the unit prompts 10-30% of individuals creating cirrhosis in five years. Treatment with pegylated interferon and ribavirin post-relocate diminishes the risk of reoccurrence to 70%.

A 2013 survey found no obvious proof with respect to whether antiviral prescription is helpful in the event that the graft becomes reinjected.

Alternative treatments

A few alternative treatments are guaranteed by their defense abilities to be useful for hepatitis C, including ginseng, milk thistle and colloidal silver. Nonetheless, no alternative treatment has been proved to improve results for hepatitis C patients, and no proof exists that elective treatments affect the virus.

Chapter 6

Diet Suggestions

There is definitely not a particular diet plan to follow assuming that you have hepatitis C, yet eating quality and healthy food — and removing food varieties that miss the mark on the parcel of healthy and nutritional benefits — is much of the time a decent spot to begin.

All that you eat and drink must be worked upon by the liver. Keeping up with appropriate nutrition can improve the strength of your liver and may try and decrease the effect of hepatitis C.

Your liver is already dealing with inflammation if you have hepatitis C. After some time, this can prompt scarring (cirrhosis) and decreased liver capability. At the end of the day, your liver is dealing with a ton. Healthy eating may help alleviate some of this stress on the liver.

What your diet ought to incorporate

Getting the right supplements is vital to your general well-being. Besides the fact that its support is needed for a good immune system, yet it likewise affects body weight the Management.

It's vital to keep your weight in a sound check, particularly in the event that you have hepatitis C. Having diabetes or being overweight can prompt hepatic steatosis, a condition brought about by high-level fat development in the liver. This can make hepatitis C harder to control. Because people who have hepatitis C are also more likely to develop type 2 diabetes, it's important to watch how much sugar you eat.

The US Branch of Horticulture's plan suggests the below for a balanced diet:

Vegetables and fruits

Vegetables and fruits supply nutrients like:

Vitamin A, C, B6, fiber, Potassium, and folate.

You ought to eat somewhere in the range of 1 to 3 cups of vegetables every day. To get the greatest scope of nutrients, differ the types of veggies you eat.

A 2013 creature examination proposed that green vegetables might be particularly useful in diminishing the unsaturated fat piece in your liver.

While buying canned vegetables, choose no-salt and no-sugar-added varieties.

Protein

Food varieties containing protein are vital. Protein helps fix and supplant liver cells harmed by hepatitis C.

<u>*Protein choices include:*</u>

Soy products, fish, chicken, nuts, seafood, eggs.

How much protein you eat everyday relies on your age, sex, and performance level.

Two to six and a half ounces of protein is usually sufficient.

Green smoothies that incorporate protein powder can assist you with hitting your protein and leafy foods targets when you're in for a short time. On the off chance that you have cirrhosis, your Dr. might prescribe a higher protein consumption to lessen your risk of muscle waste and liquid development.

Dairy

Dairy products, like milk, cheese, and yogurt, are a good source of calcium and protein. Adults who aren't lactose bigoted need somewhere in the range of 2 and 3 servings every day. This amounts to roughly one and a half tablespoons of natural cheese or one cup of milk, yogurt, or soy milk.

Whole grains

Whole grains are a great source of dietary fiber, which advances health bowels capability and decreases your risk for coronary illness or heart diseases.

<u>Whole grains include:</u>

- ➢ Whole wheat, buckwheat, or quinoa pastas
- ➢ Brown or wild rice
- ➢ Entire oats

➢ *Sprouted whole grain bread*

Whole-grain alternatives are preferable to white or refined varieties. Whole-grain are regularly higher in:

- *Vitamin B*
- *Fiber*
- *Magnesium*
- *Iron*
- *Zinc*

Eat only gluten-free grains like buckwheat, quinoa, and amaranth if you have celiac disease.

How much grain you ought to have relies upon your age, sex, and your performance level. At a neutral level, adults ought to eat around 3 to 8 ounces of grain food varieties every day. Whole-grain foods should make up at least half of those servings.

Espresso (coffee) and caffeine

Talk to your healthcare provider about including tea or coffee in your plan if you enjoy it. A little quantity of caffeine (just 100 mg) has been proved to possibly help safeguard against advanced hepatic fibrosis in men with chronic HCV infection.

More research is required and needed to entirely grasp these discoveries and their impacts on different people.

Different ingredients in food varieties are in early examinations for their likely advantages for chronic hepatitis C, like phenolic catechins from green tea and oligomeric proanthocyanidin from blueberry leaves.

Green tea has advantageous properties in everyday life as well as being an enjoyable beverage. As we learn more about its effects on hepatitis C, adding it to your routine may be beneficial.

What you ought to cut down

Calories count, so think amount as well as quality. Eating an excessive amount may prompt weight gain or obesity, which can build your diabetes risk.

Your health care provider may likewise encourage different adjustments to protect your liver, like a low-iron diet for chronic hepatitis C. The body can become overloaded with iron as a result of chronic hepatitis C, which can be harmful. These suggestions will differ depending on your medical history.

<u>*As a rule, you ought to restrict from food varieties that are:*</u>

- o *Processed*
- o *Greasy*
- o *Fatty*
- o *Frozen canned from chain restaurants*
- o *Reduce your intake of salt.*

Removing dishes that are high in sodium is particularly of great importance. Pungent food varieties can prompt water maintenance, thus raising your pulse or blood pressure. This can be risky and dangerous for individuals with cirrhosis.

Assuming your sickness is in its earliest stages, a periodic shake of the salt shaker might be fine, yet you ought to converse with your healthcare provider about how much sodium is suitable for you.

Scale back your sugar consumption

Sweet treats, when eaten too much, can prompt weight gain. To assist with remaining in good shape, you might find it supportive to enjoy occasionally as opposed to removing sugar totally. You can have your cake and eat it too in this way. Additionally, fruit is an excellent sweet option.

Tips for good dieting

<u>Things to Do:</u>

- ❖ *Make a standard eating schedule that works for you. This could be three moderate dinners daily or four to five more small meals at splatted spans.*
- ❖ *Drink six to eight glasses of water and different liquids every day*
- ❖ *Center around natural, whole and unprocessed food variety.*
- ❖ *Go natural whenever the situation allows. This can assist with restricting how much pesticides and toxins ingested through your food.*

* *Pick lean protein sources rather than fattier meats like beef.*
* *Use no-salt flavors and spices for some extra flavor.*

<u>*Don't:*</u>

* *Consume alcoholic drinks*
* *Eat more than needed to keep up with ideal wellbeing and health.*
* *Add salt to your food. .*
* *Eat a great deal of excessively processed food varieties. Depend vigorously on dietary supplements.*

Assuming you're living with hepatitis C, your nourishing necessities probably won't wander a long way from the identical nutritional guidelines, however your health care provider can give you individual benchmarks.

By and large, a decent food plan is one that emphasizes vegetables, takes out liquor, and assists you with keeping a healthy body weight. Being agile and active is useful while living with hepatitis C and as a rule, so converse with your doc about what kind of exercise is ideal for you.

Chapter 7

Caregivers Guide

There are around 3.2 million individuals all through the US who are at present living with Hepatitis C and however there will be roughly 2,200 new cases announced, specialists gauge that the number of new cases has multiplied 23 times higher. This implies that by far most of the people who are living with this disease don't realize that they are living with it, putting them at serious risk of inconveniences and putting everyone around them at extreme risk of contamination. In the event that you are a parental figure for an experiencing this casualty illness, the care that you give them can have a huge effect on their wellbeing and prosperity going forward.

At the point when somebody you love and care about has hepatitis C, you become a hepatitis C fighter right next to them even if you're a worker (home keeper,) You're in the fight with them.

Providing care responsibility can shift contingent upon the ailment of the patient. For caregivers who are assisting patients with decompensated cirrhosis, liver disease, extrahepatic conditions, or liver transplant, the needs are significantly bigger and greater.

Beat drinking and discourage alcohol.

Hepatitis C is a sickness of the liver. Liquor can prompt broad harm to the liver, including expanding the pace of liver disease's advance. On the off chance that your patient drinks liquor, urge them to stop to safeguard their liver.

Keep away from blood contamination.

Hepatitis C is a very infectious illness that can be transferred to others through contact with the blood of an already infected individual. As a caregiver, this implies that you may be at risk. Avoid potential risk by not coming in contact with your patients' blood, including wearing gloves and never sharing cups, razors, or toothbrushes with them.

Caregivers can frequently get fatigued physically, physiologically or emotionally, mentally. The caregiver should get care and support much often too. Support, and refreshments, and solving personal problematic are vital issues.

Staying balanced & avoid Burnout

In the event that a caregiver doesn't get help and care for themselves, they can't help and support the patient when required or efficiently.

<u>How caregivers can stay balanced and Avoid Burnout</u>

- ✓ *Engage in a care and support groups for Caregivers of those with liver illness.*

- ✓ *Find other people who can assist with the patient's requirements that way the obligations are shared, lighter, and more simple to deal with.*
- ✓ *Ask family, companions or healthcare services experts to help.*
- ✓ *A counseling session for the emotional support of caregiver is exceptionally useful.*
- ✓ *Take short breaks to get things done, go out with loved ones, family and friends, or work on a most loved side interest or passion can give an increase in mental refreshments. Ask a relative or companion to help for a brief time while you enjoy some time off.*
- ✓ *Always know that you are not at any point to be blamed for regarding*

what befalls the patient beyond your capacity and control.

✓ *Try not to bear loads alone. Converse with others, request help.*

✓ *On the off chance that feelings erupt, have some time off. Keep in mind, you're not godlike or a superman.*

Chapter 8

Jesus the Way Out

There's another way out of Hepatitis C: The way is called Jesus!

To be sure there's no disease, be it terminal that God can't cure. Regardless of what has held you down, Jesus speaking In Matthew 11:28 " Come to me, all you that work and are weighty loaded, and I will give you rest. Convey my burden upon you, and learn from me; for I'm meek in heart: and you will find rest unto your spirits. For my burden is extremely simple, and my weight is truly light."

Despite what you are going through Jesus can help you on the off chance that you can accept and believe in him.

In any case, to do that, you must have received him into your life. In the event that you have not received Jesus Christ, say this prayers:

"Dear Jesus, I acknowledge that I am a sinner. I acknowledge that you did die on the cross for my avocation and justification. Thusly I acknowledge you as my Ruler, lord and personal savior from now on. Also, I declare and pronounce that the power of transgression, the force of Satan, the

force of agony is broken over my life for I'm in Christ now. So be it"

The best supernatural miracle is about to happen because you believe him. Entrust God with your healing and each and every other issue.

Here are a few bible verses that could help you;

Isaiah 38:16-17, Isaiah 40:29, Isaiah 57:18-29, Jeremiah 30:17 „Jeremiah 33:6, Matthew 11:28... .. Rush to Jesus now!!!

Simply in case you really need guidance, reach out through this mail - will394560@gmail.com

God bless you!

9 798880 329342